KETOGENIC DIET

Your Guide To Lose Weight

With A Low Carb And

High Fat Diet

I0435388

Kris Tyson

The trademarks that are used are without any consent, and the publication of the trademark is without permission or backing by the trademark owner. All trademarks and brands within this book are for clarifying purposes only and are the owned by the owners themselves, not affiliated with this document.

Table of Contents

MAKE SURE TO CHECK OUT MY OTHER BOOKS:

- Beginner's Guide to the Paleo Diet: A Simple Start to Achieving Optimal Health and Weight Loss through the Original Human Diet + 35 FREE RECIPES (FREE)
- Ketogenic Diet: A Beginner's Guide to the Ketogenic Diet (Low Carb, High Fat Diet to Lose Weight and Live a Healthy Lifestyle + 35 Bonus recipes

- Low Carb Diet Recipes: 90 Days of Low Carbohydrate Recipes

Introduction: What exactly is a Ketogenic Diet?

Ketogenic diet was visualized out of "Ketosis", a procedure through which your body is ready to separate more fat into free-fatty acid, as a result of utilizing low carb diet, for example, Ketogenic diet. The fatty acids and ketones discharged as an aftereffect of this break down will deliver more energy for the body.

Free fatty acids and Ketones are regularly released concurrently during the breakdown of fats in the body, and with more ketones and fatty acids in the body, your body will have more energy to burn as fuel. Normally, the body burns Glucose-a produce discharged from the breakdown of sugar from carbohydrates (carb). At the point when your body blazes Glucose as a type of energy, the stored fat in your body remain , however when the body burns fatty acids and Ketones when there are less adequate glucose (as a consequence of utilizing ketogenic diet), the body will rapidly go through store fat in essential organs, for example, the liver , and the muscles. The general impact of this procedure is that you get in shape quickly and still find sufficient energy to maintain your every day exercises.

You have to observe that, the body can just burn any energy source present, and with a low carb ketogenic diet, there is a small amount of carb present, hence the body will turn to fat as a source of fuel.

When you utilize high carb diet, the body burns the carbs as energy, however the way that there is excess means the body needs to store them some place (the muscles and organs). At the point when excess carbs are not spent as needs to be, they will make you put on more weight quickly, particularly when you are not active. With a Ketogenic diet, you feel more fulfilled immediately when you eat, therefore you consume significantly less carbs that might in the end get separated and store as fat in your organs and muscles. Ketogenic diet will offer the body some assistance with using up more stored energy. With the consumption up of more energy, your Insulin hormones turn out to be more synchronized.

Ketogenic diet is not a magical weight loss formula; however, you have to perceive that calories matter, with regards to weight loss. With a specific end goal to get more fitness and stay healthy, there must be an energy balance in your body, and this balance must be made when you utilize more energy than you consume. Ketogenic diet works in two ways; first it doesn't place you in any starving mode, besides, it makes a net-equalization in the way you ingest and consume energy.

On the off chance that your body gets all of its energy from the diet you eat on regular schedule, it turns out to be practically difficult to quantify the amount of energy you consume, however when you are sure that your ketogenic diet has less carbs, and a greater amount of different supplements, it is simpler to identify whether you are making a net-balance of energy. While a few individuals eat while they are hungry, and consume what they have to wind up fulfilled, others do eat without bounds limit, regardless of whether they are very hungry or not. When you eat not to get full, it is simpler to get more fitness.

The fundamental guideline of Ketogenic diet is that you should avoid starchy foods (most particularly high carb prepared foods), grains, tubers and sugars. These ought to be replaced with meat, fertile greens, over the ground vegetables, dairy, nuts and seeds, avocado, berries and a few fats, for example, cream cheddar and coconut oil.

Chapter 1: The Importance and benefits of a low carb diet

In opposition to the accept by numerous that Ketogenic diets will bring cholesterol levels in the body in view of its low carb and high protein and fat parts, the situation is totally different. Since the body will now blaze more fat from the diets, the amount of fat ingested will be too little, as long as the fundamental source of energy is not carb but rather fat. Ketogenic diet drives the body to depend on fat for its essential source of energy, rather of carbs. Here are some different advantages of Ketogenic diet worth saying;

- **Removes sugar yearnings and unnecessary hunger**

One of the fundamental reasons individuals think that it's hard to get more fitness is that they can't control their craving for food. Ketogenic diets offer you some assistance with controlling your dietary pattern because a diet rich in fat can be exceptionally fulfilling inside a short time period. When you begin a Ketogenic diet, you will see that occasionally, you simply lose interest in eating, and this could be the most astonishing part, particularly when you battle with some issues of food addiction.

- **Speeds up weight loss and helps to build more lean muscle**

Studies have demonstrated that individual placed on low carb diets lose more than double the weight of those put on low fat diet over the same timeframe. One of the fundamental explanations behind this impact is that low carb dieters regularly end up disposing of water rapidly from their bodies, and the way that a lower insulin level will drive the kidney to shed excess sodium, in their bodies, consequently prompting fast loss in weight even inside of a short timeframe. When you achieve your desired weight level, you might include a healthy carb, back to your every day calorie utilization.

- Most fat lost during Ketogenic dieting will originate from abdominal cavity

One of the most fortunate things about Ketogenic dieting is that a large portion of the fat lost originates from the most difficult parts of the body, most particularly the abdominal cavity. The way fat is stored in your body will decide how it influences your health. On the off chance that the greater part of the fat in your body is circulated in your mid-section, particularly where fundamental organs are found, then your health is at risk. Having extreme fat in the body can trigger insulin resistance, inflammation, and some different serious illnesses. Subsequently, a ketogenic diet is best for you if you battle with a fat store in your stomach region.

- Ketogenic diet decreases Triglycerides levels in the body

Triglycerides have been connected with different heart infections, and the primary driver of triglycerides in the body is carbohydrates, particularly those from simple sugars. At the point when compared with different diets, low carb ketogenic diets will viably decrease triglycerides by as much as 65% in the blood.

- It builds HDL cholesterol levels in the body

HDL cholesterol, likewise known a High Density Lipoprotein is normally referred to good cholesterol, which is healthy for the body. They are lipoproteins that bear cholesterol the blood while LDL or bad cholesterol is often carried from the liver to other remains of the body, where they can be reused or discharged from the body at any time. HDL carries bad cholesterol from the body and the liver hence they can be immediately removed. One of the most ideal methods for expanding your blood's HDL level is to consume low carb Ketogenic diet, it lower triglyceride arrangement and keep your essential organs healthier.

- Reduces glucose levels and controls Insulin resilience

One of the best news for diabetes patients is that Ketogenic diets are fit for diminishing glucose levels. When you eat high carb foods, they will be separated into basic sugars, particularly in the digestive tracts. At the point when simple sugars enter the circulation system, they rapidly raise glucose levels and insulin sensitivity. Healthy individuals will have rapidly insulin controlling their glucose level however diabetic patients may not be as fortunate and a sharp increment in sugar in the blood might bring about damage.

When you create insulin resistance, it implies your body cells don't get adequate measure of insulin to carry glucose into cells however when you consume a low carb ketogenic diet, you will kill the requirement for excess insulin, and your glucose gets to be normalized.

- It minimizes pulse

Having elevated blood pressure all the time will become obvious eventually your dangers to a few sorts of infections, including heart diseases, kidney failure and stroke. Low carb diets have been found through clinical studies to bring down the chances to develop these diseases.

- Low carb diets wipe out different metabolic disorders

Metabolic disorders have been connected with a few different other diseases, for example, diabetes and heart diseases. Metabolic disorders are actually side effects of different issue, for example; stomach problem, hypertension, high glucose levels, and High triglycerides. The good news is that low carb diet will extraordinarily enhance these indications once you begin taking ketogenic diets.

- Provides remedial impacts for different brain issues

However, Glucose is essential for a healthy and practical brain, yet a few sections of the mind can just blaze glucose and when we don't eat adequate carbs, the liver will deliver more glucose from protein. A few sections of the mind likewise burn ketones, particularly when you are in a starving mode or when you consume low carb diets. Ketogenic diets have been utilized for quite a long time to offer children some assistance with suffering from epilepsy and when they are not reacting to ordinary medicines.

- Boosts immunity

The overall result of consuming low carb diets is that the immunity of the entire system is strengthened against the harmful diseases.

Chapter 2: How does Ketogenic diet work to help you lose weight fast?

What you are intended to eat will influence whether you get in shape or not. Early people were accustomed to eating through chasing, they eat consumable foods, fish and meat with almost no starch, nonetheless, the present day world has prompted the revelation of handled food, including pasta, bread, potato and rice. With mechanical upsets, white flour and pure sugar were delivered and these are moderate nutritions that the body has not changed by.

The issue with sugar and starch is that all edible carbs are separated into simple sugars, in the small digestive tract, before the sugar is ingested into the circulatory system. This prompts a fast increment in blood glucose level and the discharge of more insulin hormones. Insulin hormones are discharged from the pancreas, and they typically prevent copying of fat while putting away supplements in fat cells. Before long, when insulin has been discharged into the circulatory system, you might start feeling hungry again, on the grounds that there is an apparent lack of supplements in the blood, and as of right now, the vast majority will consider eating another significant dinner this is the place the endless loop of weight addition begins.

Then again, the utilization of low carb ketogenic diet will deliver much lower blood glucose, in this way prompting a lower measure of insulin discharged into the blood. This will, in the long run, expand the measure of fats put away in your fat stores (counting the liver and kidney), which will accelerate the fat-burning procedure. Bulky individual or those with abundance fat around the stomach area can depend on Ketogenic diets for rapid blazing of fat.

Ketogenic diet gives weight loss without hunger

Since Ketogenic diet makes it much simpler for the body to make utilization of its fat stores because the arrival of such fat stores won't be obstructed by Insulin hormones. This might conceivably be one reason eating high fat diets deliver longer satiety or diminish sustenance cravings, than eating high starch foods. Thus, there is no compelling reason to begin adding calories. On the off chance that you don't trust this weight loss process, simply attempt Ketogenic diets for 1 week and you will be convinced without any doubt.

What's in store for your first week of consuming Ketogenic diets

If you quit eating sugar and starch unexpectedly, you might witness some slight symptoms as your body rapidly modifies. For a great many people, the symptoms might be smooth, and might keep going for the only a couple of days. A percentage of the underlying symptoms might incorporate;

- Dizziness,

- Headache,

-Fatigue,

- Irritability, and

- Heart diseases.

As your body adjusts to the new health routine, the symptoms will progressively die down. One of the ideal approaches to minimize these slight reactions is to build your water consumption or somewhat expand your salt admission. The primary explanation behind this stride is that high carb foods regularly expand the water-maintenance limit of the body, and when you begin expending low carb ketogenic diets, you will begin losing more water, particularly from essential organs, for example, the kidneys-this might in the result in lack of hydration and low salt levels(most particularly among your initial couple of days of beginning ketogenic diet).

To offer your body, some assistance with adjusting step by step diminishes the entry of starches more than a couple of weeks so as to minimize symptoms of such diets. For a few individuals, simply doing the weight loss program immediately is an ideal approach to take as their bodies will, in the end, get up to speed paying little respect to the symptoms they need to succeed.

Chapter 3: Preparing for Ketogenic diet weight loss program

Get ready for Ketogenic diet weight loss treatment ought to be positive, the reason being that the more you set up your body, the snappier your body can change the system and the more health advantages you can get from it.

In a perfect world, the planning for Ketogenic diet weight loss system ought to begin between 2-7 days before you start. You have to make a schedule of the foods you will use and ensure that you make unique menus, to guarantee that you don't stick to one routine, and the routine does not get to be exhausting. Although making a plan, making a period table of what you will eat will offer you some assistance with preparing ahead without getting adhered to the same food.

While the utilization of activities may not be entirely prescribed, but rather it is perfect to get rid of an inactive way of life particularly on the off chance that you work requires that you sit in a position for a few hours. There are low effect and fun practices you can begin honing before you start despite among the ketogenic diet program. Low effect activities, for example, swimming and cycling are suggested however not entirely forced.

Just before you initiate the Ketogenic diet program, you have to ensure that you start taking out some of your normal foods, these are overwhelmingly involved sugar and handled foods. Nutrition, for example, sugar, white bread, sugary refreshments, grains and heated items and other overwhelming carb diets must be wiped out before the beginning of Ketogenic diet.

You have to guarantee that your body is detoxified to accelerate your weight loss process amid Ketogenic dieting. Thus, it is suggested that you expend various leafy foods, to expand your fiber allow and kill wastes and acids. Keep in mind; a lower harmful level will encourage your weight loss. If possible, you ought to perform some squeezes through the utilization of foods grown from the ground smoothies.

Since water-maintenance limits are brought down between ketogenic dieting, it is necessary that you wipe out liquor and juiced drinks that will make you lose more water and feel got dried out.

Continuously remember that setting up your body for ketogenic dieting will accelerate your weight loss length of time and make you accomplish significantly more advantages.

Chapter 4: What to eat and what to avoid when feasting on Ketogenic diet

The Ketogenic diet methodology is straightforward and simple; eat genuine foods and avoid high carbs. You have to consider eating genuine and nutritious foods, for example, eggs, meat, nuts, dairy, vegetables and organic products. From your shopping rundown to dietary pattern, Ketogenic diets must go through everything. Here is a manual for what you need to consume as Ketogenic diet;

#1 Meat – numerous sorts of meats are prescribed, these incorporate; hamburger, fun meat, pork, turkey, and chicken. Ensure you blend the greasy part of the meat with the incline and skin bit. In the event that possible, attempt however much as could reasonably be expected to consume naturally raised creatures, and ensure the meat is appropriately cleaned before cooking.

#2 Fish-These include a wide range of fishes, and shellfish. Unique decisions include; Salmon, Herring, and Mackerel, however attempt as much as could reasonably be expected to refrain from breading.

#3 Eggs-a wide range of eggs can be used yet all the more critically, naturally raised poultry eggs are prescribed. Eggs consumed as Ketogenic diet can be boiled, scorch or made as Omelets.

#4 Natural fats and high fat sauces-You might consider

cooking your dinners with spread and cream since they make your foods taste great and can make you feel satisfied the more. Hollandaise sauce is likewise suggested, however, you should check every one of the fixings utilized as a part of making the sauce or essentially make one independent from anyone else. You can likewise make utilization of coconut or olive oil for cooking and different types of cooking oils.

#5 Vegetables grow over the ground – Vegetables that grow over the ground are wonderful wellsprings of vital minerals and vitamins. You need to consider vegetables, for example, Cauliflower, Cabbage, Brussels grows, Broccoli, Eggplant, Asparagus, Olives, Zucchini, mushrooms, spinach, Lettuce, Avocado, Cucumber, Peppers, Onions, and Tomatoes.

#6 Dairy Foods - Dairy items must be chosen on the off chance that you are not oversensitive to a few foods, for example, milk. On the off chance that you have lactose intolerance, then you have to consider conversing with your specialist about option decisions you can make. For dairy items you should choose full-fat or medium-fat choices, for example, cream (around 40% fat), spread, Greek Yogurt, Turkish yogurt, High-fat cheddar, acrid cream, and Greek cheddar. You should be careful with the utilization of skimmed and consistent milk since they contain milk sugar. Correspondingly, attempt as much as could be expected to stay away from seasoned, low fat items, and sugary nourishments.

#7 Nuts and seeds-these are very nutritious foodss with loads of protein. They can be your best mates when watching the TV, along these lines they are great substitutions for confections and other unhealthy sugary snacks. A percentage of the best nuts and seeds you have to consider add in; peanuts, and groundnuts.

#8 Berries-Berries are alright however should be consumed with some limit, most particularly in the event that you are delicate to them. Berries are awesome and delicious when overcome with whipped cream. There are no restrictions to the decisions of berries you can consider; strawberries, Cranberries, blueberries and blackberries are a part of the best.

#9: fluids water is highly suggested, it keeps you hydrated despite the fact that your body's water maintenance limit might be brought down while consuming Ketogenic diet. Water will maintain your program by transporting supplements to all parts of your body. Attempt as much as could reasonably be expected to keep away from energized drinks since they are diuretic in nature and you might need to urinate constantly this imply you will stay got dried out.

Attempt however as much as could reasonably be expected to read carefully the marks of all nourishment things before purchasing them at the supermarkets. The dependable guideline here is that your diet ought to be 5% or less carbs.

What to maintain a strategic distance from in Ketogenic dieting

Ketogenic diet works best to offer you some assistance with losing weight on the off chance that you stay with prescribed sustenance classes as highlighted previously. You should attempt as much as you can to stay away from or to a great extent include the following;

#1 Sugar-This is the most noticeably awful of all of them. Sugars come in various forms, in this manner you should keep away from foods and refreshments, for example, carbonated soda pops, Buns, cakes, baked goods, sugar breakfast oats, cakes, and frozen yogurt. On the off chance that possible, attempt as much as you need to keep away from simulated sweeteners.

#2 Starch-Just like handled sugars, starches likewise contain high carbs and must be maintained a possible distance from it if possible. Bland foods to keep away from include; Pasta, Potatoes, Bread, rice, porridge, French fries, Potato chips, and muesli. Be careful with vegetables and lentils since they contain a definite amount of starch, similarly entire grain foods might contain shrouded sugar. If you should consume root vegetables, then you have to practice control.

#3-Margarine-Margarines are prepared with some engineered materials, including hydrogen, in this way they contain a high measure of Omega-6 unsaturated fats – these have no health advantages although the way that they taste so terrible. Margarine has been clinically connected to a few diseases, including compounding of asthma side effects, incendiary infections and the intensifying of a few other nutrition hypersensitivities.

#4 Alcoholic drinks - Though red and white wine might be consumed cautiously, they might contain hidden sugars that should be maintained a strategic distance from. Brew contains carbs that can be promptly assimilated. Consequently, they should be maintained a strategic distance at any cost.

#5 Fruits - If you should consume organic products, they should be half un-aged ones, and the reason being that ready natural products are sweet and contains bunches of sugar. You need to regard ready organic products as regular types of confections; along these lines, they should be consumed carefully.

Now and again, you might consider eating dull chocolate since they are comprised of 70% cocoa. If you should consume some liquor, then you should evade general dry wine (red or white), whiskey, mixed drinks, schnaps or vodka that contains sugar. You should drink water or tea without sugar, and if you should take espresso, then try the one with full fat cream.

On the off chance that you have an adequate measure of time to work-out, particularly at a young hour in the morning, then you need to go for low-affect works out. Some cardio workouts, weight-lifting and other extending activities can keep you going and rev up your digestion system for whatever is left of the day.

Chapter 5: Ketogenic diet protocols (rules you must follow to ensure success)

Ketogenic diet conventions or belief directs the appropriate measure of every nourishment (most extreme), that should be included at once in your dinners. It additionally discloses how to settle on your decisions and stick to the low carb standards of the diet. Here are Ketogenic diet conventionss you have to take after;

Creature item conventions

- Meat and fish give 0-net carbs and must not surpass 150g/serving

- Eggs give around 1.4 net carbs (grams), this must not surpass 150g for every serving,

- The full fat cream gives 1.6 net carb; it must not surpass ¼ a glass or 60ml for every serving.

- Cheese (hard), gives 0.4 net carbs and must not surpass 30g for every serving.

- Cream cheddar (full fat), gives 1.6 net carbs, and must not surpass ¼ glass or 50g for every serving.

Vegetables - Protocol

- Vegetables, for example, Lettuce, Asparagus, Cucumber,

Cooked Spinach, Cabbage, Celery stalk, Cauliflower, Chopped Broccoli, and Dark leaf kale gives somewhere around 1.2 and 6.4 net carb (grams) and must not surpass 150g for each serving.

- Vegetables, for example, Brown or white mushrooms, Onions Tomatoes, green or red pepper, green beans, garlic and cut white onions give somewhere around 1.2 and 5.9 net calories(grams), these must not surpass ½ container or 50grams for each serving.

Organic products Protocol

- Sliced strawberries produce up to 4.7(grams) and must not surpass ½ a glass or 85g for each serving.

- Raspberries produce around 3.3 net carbs, and must not surpass ½ a glass or 62g for each serving.

- Blackberries give somewhere in the range of 3.2 net carbs and must not surpass ½ a glass or 72 grams for every serving.

- Blueberries contain somewhere in the range of 8.9 net carbs, and must not surpass ½ a glass or 74g for every serving.

- Avocado gives around 3.7 net carbs and ought to be pierced into a normal of 200g for every serving.

Nuts and Seeds – Protocol

- Almonds give around 2.7 net carbs(grams), and must not surpass 30g for every serving.

- Hazelnuts give around 2 net carbs (grams) and must not surpass 30g for every serving.

- Walnuts give nearly 2 net carbs (grams), and must not

surpass 30g for each serving.

- Other seeds, for example, China seeds, sunflower seeds, Pumpkin seeds, and pecans give somewhere around 0.4 and 7.6 net carbs (grams), and must not surpass a tablespoon or 30g for each serving.

Fixings and others - conventions

- Condiments, sauce and other related additional items, for example, sugar-free Almond milk, creamed coconut milk, olive oil, mustard, tomato puree, apple juice vinegar, dull chocolate, flax dinner, stevia, dry red or white wine, gives somewhere around 0.1 and 5.7 net carbs, and must not be incorporated at levels of between ¼ container (60mls), and 1 glass for each serving.

Fish, Meat, and Sea nourishments conventions

- You ought to think about eating a fish that was gotten; these include; Cod, Flounder, Halibut, fish, Salmon, Trout, and mackerel. Shellfishes you can consume include; Scallops, Lobsters, Clams, Crab, mussels, and squids. Fishes can make up the heft of your diet, and it is suggested that you eat at the very least 250g for every serving.

- Meat, for example, Veal, Hamburger, goat, wild diversion and any naturally sustained creature are the best since they contain higher unsaturated fat tally. This ought to be an essential part of your Ketogenic diet and should be incorporated at the very least 400g a day.

- Pork might be incorporated or substituted with meat and

fish. You have to go for Pork cleaves, pork loins, and ham (attempt as much as possible to keep away from any additional sugar to the ham). Pork ought to be included in your diet at not more than 150g at once.

- Bacon and hotdog are perfect, however, try as much as possible to maintain a strategic distance from any additional sugars in the ham. Bacon and hotdog ought to be included at no more than 100g for each serving.

- Peanut margarine Natural nutty spread is the best, yet you have to practice carefully since they contain high measure of omega 6 and carbs. A perfect alternative is Macadamia nut spread. Nutty spread need to be carefully utilized as a part of any Ketogenic diet.

General Ketogenic diet conventions

- The general conventions of Ketogenic dieting is that at least 80% of your diet need to include healthy fat while 15% need to contain key proteins, vitamins and minerals. Any Ketogenic diet must contain under 5 % of carbs because you need to eliminate starches and compel your body to burn fat as energy.

- Depending on the term you need to go, it is perfect to begin with a 72-hour Ketogenic diet straight, whereby you have a day or 2 to set up your body and after that begin the Ketogenic diet on the third day through to the fifth day. One of the advantages of having a slow Ketogenic diet routine is that it offers your body some assistance with recovering rapidly from any impact that may come about because of authorizing Ketogenic diets and getting a break after every 3 days is an ideal method for accomplishing this.

- Try as much as possible to substitute the foods in each

prescribed classification, to guarantee that you don't get exhausted eating the same sustenance constantly. For example, you can consume fish and pork today, and then eat a greater amount of hamburger and chicken the next day.

- Being active between your Ketogenic diet routine is prescribed, however, you don't need to be included in high effect works out. A moderate effect activity is prescribed to offer you some assistance with burning fat. The best activities for Ketogenic diet is performed at a young hour in the morning, before 7 AM and late at night, around 6-7PM. Low effect practices prescribed for Ketogenic diet routine include; extending works out, cardio workouts, weight lifting, high impact exercise, cycling, swimming and lively strolling.

Chapter 6: Ketogenic diet mistakes to avoid

Keeping in mind the end goal to get thinner through the utilization of Ketogenic diets, there are sure missteps you should know about, these mix-ups are highlighted underneath;

Rules #1: Not recharging your body's Sodium levels

One of the impacts of expending a low carb Ketogenic diet is that it decreases Insulin levels, and one of the fundamental elements of Insulin is to direct cells to store fats. Another significant capacity of insulin is to alert the kidneys to hold immovably unto its sodium. When you use low-fat Ketogenic diets for quite a while, your insulin levels go low and your body loses more sodium close by the generous measure of water-this is one reason the vast majority frequently dispose of bloating even inside of the initial 24 hours of expending low carb diets.

You have to remember that sodium is a key electrolyte in the body, and the overabundance shedding of it from the kidneys can make a serious health hazard. The overabundance shedding of sodium might bring about some slight issues, for example, tipsiness, cerebral pains, uniform, and clogging, particularly among an initial couple of days of Ketogenic dieting. The best way to stay away from this issue is to increment marginally, your salt admission (you might likewise consume juices now and again). This will offer you some assistance with increasing your sodium level fundamentally.

Rules #2 expending an excessive amount of protein

You have to remember that the fundamental objective of low

carb Ketogenic diet is to expend healthy fat and not protein, as we as a whole realize that protein is an essentially miniaturized scale supplement that can enhance satiety while expanding fat burning .with this trust, more protein should lead to weight loss and enhance radically, your body creation, yet the issue is that low carb dieters who consume incline creature proteins will wind up eating a lot of it and when you eat more protein than your body needs, your body will change over the abundance into Glucose and this will keep your body from getting into "Ketosis" stage. Your body won't blaze adequate fat to make you get more fit until it enters the Ketosis stage, in this manner you have to restrain your protein utilization to 10% or less of your aggregate diet. A perfect defined Ketogenic diet need to have low carb with high fat and direct protein

Rules #3: Consuming more carbs than prescribed levels

A few individuals don't stay with the prescribed <5% carb for Ketogenic diet. Some might be befuddled at what precisely constitute a low carb diet by assessing that anything less than 150g of carb a day is "low carb." There might be no issue in the event that you get 150g of carbs a day from natural starch foods, however, fast beverages, for example, carbonated sodas and ready organic products can pointedly expand your carb consumption, making you take more than would normally be appropriate and this can prompt an expansion in blood glucose, with a resultant impact of increment in insulin levels. It might take some experimentation before you can find how to measure your carb levels, yet attempt to restrict it to 50-100g a day and pick healthy sources suggested in above sections.

Rules #4 Not being tolerant

Low carb Ketogenic diet is not a "snappy" weight loss program that will make you lose fat quickly, it takes some devotion and textures to make it work for you. Individuals regularly get into hindrances when they expect a lot inside of a short timeframe. There is one thing you have to understand about ketogenic diets. First, your body was intended to burn specially carbs rather than fat, particularly when carbs are accessible. In this way, if you make carbs accessible, that is the thing that your body will blaze. If you radically lessen your carb entry, your body will naturally move to another wellspring of energy, as a rule, fats. The fat that your body separates must come either from your diet or the stored fats in your body.

Full adjustment of the body to low carb Ketogenic diet might take a couple of days and weeks yet it will in the end yield comes about once your body has moved the center to burning fat. You should be patient to take advantage from low carb ketogenic diets.

Rules #5: Being hesitant to eat fat (eating low-fat diets)

Generalization masterminds will make you trust that eating fat is terrible, and we as a whole have been advised to dependably maintain a strategic distance from fat since we were little, yet now that reality has been uncovered through Ketogenic diets, you are currently mindful that an ideal approach to get thinner is to switch your body into a fat-burning mode, rather than carb-blazing mode. Despite the fact that it is perfect to maintain a strategic distance from awful cholesterol, including those found in vegetable oils and quick nourishments, these fats might build your chances of creating aggravation and wouldn't help your weight loss either. Try as much as possible to supplant vegetable oil with coconut oil, bacon oil, and margarine.

Rules #6: Try to force too numerous progressions on the double

You have to distinguish that some addictive ways of life can be extremely troublesome and test to change. For example attempting to dump a stationary way of life loaded with the utilization of garbage nourishments to a totally Ketogenic way of life of low carb ought to take a time of arrangement since you would prefer not to put an excess of weight on your body inside of a short timeframe. Measurements and looks into have demonstrated that people who get sufficiently ready before the beginning of ketogenic diets regularly wind up making the greatest achievements of weight loss.

Rules #7: Not coordinating your diets enough

Blending and coordinating diets is one of an ideal methods for getting a charge out of low carb ketogenic diet and shedding pounds. You have to make a period table and substitute comparative nourishment parts for each other, to make a flawless and well adjust schedule that you can stick to without getting exhausted rapidly. You have to guarantee that utilization of comparative foods are exchanged inside of days separated and ensure you expend as much water as your body can hold.

Attempt as much as you can to stay away from every single of these slip-ups on the off chance that you need to get the best from your low carb Ketogenic diet for weight loss.

Chapter 7: Some of the best Ketogenic diet recipes you should consider

This section will control you on a percentage of the best low carb Ketogenic formulas and also proposals on the best way to settle on the ideal decisions for your breakfast, lunch and supper;

Breakfast formula recommendations

- Omelet,

- Eggs and Bacon,

- Coffee with cream,

- Boiled eggs with a container of mackerel,

- Boiled eggs with mayonnaise and spread,

- Sour cream with avocado and salmon,

- Oopsie bread with sandwich,

- Butter with cheddar,

- Boiled eggs, crushed with margarin, salt, pepper, and chives (hacked),

- Brie cheddar with some salami or ham, and

- High-fat yogurt presented with seeds, nuts or berries.

Lunch and Dinner recommendations

- Fish, meat or chicken dishes presented with vegetables with a rich full-fat sauce. You can likewise consider different options for potatoes, including; Cauliflower.

- Stews, dishes, and soups with some low-carb fixings.

- Consume however much water as could reasonably be expected. You might drink a glass of wine so often, however, attempt as much as you can to stay away from the brew.

Snacks

Your snacks ought to by, and large contain low carb fixings with high fats and respectably low protein. You might no more need to nibble as a result of the satisfying force of fat. The vast majority who enjoy low carb Ketogenic diet are alright with 2 or 3 suppers a day, however, on the off chance that you have to nibble, you can consider the following;

- Olives,

- Nuts,

- Rolled-up ham or cheddar with some vegetable (you might spread margarine or cheddar on the ham).

- A bit of Greek cheddar,

- Canned mackerel with some tomato sauce, and

- A boiled egg.

Attempt as much as you can to supplant potato chips with nuts and olives. On the off chance that regardless you get hungry in the middle of your dinners, then you are most likely not sufficiently consuming fat in your customary suppers.

You're shopping list as an amateur to Ketogenic diet

You ought to consider taking this rundown to a market when shopping and planning for Ketogenic diet;

- Heavy cream (around 40% fat),

- Butter,

- Sour cream (full fat),

- Meat (this could be minced, stew pieces, steaks or filets),

- Bacon,

- Eggs,

- Fish (consider purchasing greasy fishes like mackerel and salmon),

- High-fat cheddar,

- Turkish Yogurt (contains around 10% fat),

- Vegetables that grow over the ground (including cabbage,

cauliflower, Brussels sprouts, and kale),

- Olive oil,

- Avocados,

- Nuts,

- Olives, and

- Frozen vegetables, for example, Wok Vegetables and Broccoli.

Simple approaches to cooking some low carb Ketogenic diets

#1 cooking your eggs

- Gently put your eggs in some icy water and convey to bubbling at either 4 minutes of delicate bubbling or 8 minutes of hard bubbling. Peel the eggs and enjoy with your most loved mayonnaise.

- Fry your eggs in some spread on one or both sides, and then include some salt and pepper.

- Melt some spread in a skillet and include some 2-3 eggs and after that 3 tablespoons of overwhelming cream. Include your salt and pepper, and mix the blend until legitimately done. Include a few chives alongside ground cheddar on top and after that serve new with some fricasseed bacon.

- Create a player of omelet with around 3 eggs and 3 tablespoons of cream, and afterward include your flavors and salt. Liquefy a few spoons of spread in the griddle, and after that pour in the omelet player. You can fill the strong upper surface with some low carb regards, for example, cheddar or mushrooms.

#2 Making Oopsies

Oopsies are low carb different options for bread. Oopsies is a sort of bread with no carbs, these sorts of bread can likewise be consumed in various ways. You can make upwards of 6 Oopsies at once, relying upon their sizes. The fixings you have to make your Oopsies are;

- 100grams of cream cheddar,

- A squeeze of salt,

- 3 eggs,

- ½ tablespoon of Psyllium seed husks (optional), and

- ½ teaspoon of heating powder (discretionary)

Planning

- Separate the egg yolk from the egg white in various dishes,

- Gently whipped the egg white with the squeeze of salt, until the blend turns out to be firm, and that implies you ought to have the capacity to turn the blow away without the development of the egg white inside.

- Gently blend the egg yolk with the cream cheddar and you can likewise include the Psyllium seed husk with heating powder, in case you like.

- Slightly overlap the egg white into the egg yolk blend while securing the air inside the egg whites.

- Create 6 or more Oopsies on the preparing plate, and heat them on the stove at temperatures of around 300 degrees Fahrenheit. Ensure they turn brilliant before evacuating them.

- Have your low-calorie Oopsie as a sandwich or as a sausage, bun or ground sirloin sandwich. You can likewise include a few seeds them before heating them (sesame or sunflower seeds are more ideal). You can likewise include some whipped cream as a layer and enjoy the scrumptious taste.

Rather than high carb potatoes, rice and pasta, you ought to consider having squashed cauliflower, plates of mixed greens, bubbled broccoli, Vegetables au gratin, vegetables stewed in some cream (for the case, Spinach in cream), and Avocado. For your nibble treats, you ought to consider having blended nuts, vegetables with plunges, frankfurter (cut into pieces and after that additional to some cheddar and some toothpick stick through them), Cream cheddar roll (set up this by rolling some cream cheddar in some salami, alongside air-dried ham or a few cuts of cucumber). You can likewise devour olives if you can't get ready different snacks specified here.

Chapter 8: Frequently asked questions (FAQs) on Ketogenic diet

As great a low carb ketogenic diet may be, with regards to shedding pounds, and building incline muscles, a few individuals still kick befuddled about getting off with the treatment. Here are a few responses to basic inquiries asked on Low Carb Ketogenic;

Question # 1: How dependable is low carb ketogenic diet for weight loss?

Answer: with regards to low carb Ketogenic diet, your odds of getting in shape are high, given you stick the diet organization and conventions (that is more than 90% fat, and under 5% carb). Clinical trials have demonstrated that Low carb ketogenic diet has the most noteworthy odds of helping weight loss since it switches the body into a fat-blazing mode as opposed to carb-burning mode.

Question #2: wouldn't greasy foods make me gain more weight?

No! For, whatever length of time that you pick the right greasy foods suggested in this book and you guarantee that you consume less than 5% carbs in every dinner. The principle target of low carb ketogenic diet is to switch your body into a fat-burning mode. However your body is accustomed to blazing high carbs for energy, yet when there are practically no put away carbs in the body or from your diet, the body will naturally burn stored fat.

Question #3: what amount of fat is sufficient for Ketogenic diet?

From previous parts of this book, it is prescribed that at least 150g of fish, chicken, pork, poultry and other suggested fat source ought to be included into every dinner. So also, the suggested measure of other fat sources must be kept up to guarantee that you get the required measure of fat to help your weight loss.

Question #4: Do I have to quick intermittently with Ketogenic diet?

There is no requirement for discontinuous fasting when taking Ketogenic diets for weight loss, the way that high-fat foods give high satiety implies you will have the capacity to control your voracity for nourishment, and you might, in the end, avoid a few dinners and even disregard eating.

Question #5: How imperative is calorie consumption in Ketogenic diet?

There are no strict calorie confinements with low carb ketogenic diets. However, you have to stay with the 90% fat and <5% carb guideline. In spite of the fact that it is perfect to stay with under 1,800 calories a day for men and under 1,500 calories for ladies a day, these calorie limitations won't be successful if you don't stay with the 90% fat substance principle. You ought to incorporate the huge measure of protein and also vitamin and mineral sources similarly yet the diet must be prevalently fats and oils.

Question #6: imagine a scenario where I break the low carb guideline.

Once in a while breaking the principles of low carb ketogenic diet must not prevent you from proceeding with the treatment. You have to remember that the outcomes might be moderate in the first place yet when your body has completely exchanged into fat-burning mode, you will begin profiting thereof as your body seems slimmer and lighter and you have more incline muscles.

Question #7: How soon will I begin having results with low carb ketogenic diet?

Answer: You can begin accomplishing results from low carb ketogenic diet in as meager as 24-48 hours, everything relies on upon your underlying body weight and also your body organization and digestion system. It might take the length of 7 to 14 days for a few individuals to begin getting results, staying with the conventions is the most imperative thing. If you have abundance weight, you unquestionably require a more extended time to accomplish your primary objective. For novices, it is suggested that you stay with a couple of weeks of low carb ketogenic diet at once.

Question 8: what is the appropriate measure of weight loss I ought to anticipate from Ketogenic diet?

The measure of weight you can lose through low carb Ketogenic diet will rely on upon how well you stay with the conventions and for to what extent you take after the routine. People who stay with low carb Ketogenic diet for more than 3 months accomplish the best results. Thus, people who enjoy with low to direct effect can expand their rate of getting thinner by as much as half since they assemble incline muscles rapidly, and these supplant the fats being blazed.

Question 9: Are there any reactions of low carb ketogenic diets?

There might be some slight symptoms toward the start of low carb ketogenic dieting; these might incorporate, cerebral pains, tipsiness and lack of hydration. The purpose behind these reactions is that the body is attempting to change by the exchanging of its digestion system from carb-blazing to fat-burning mode. Not everybody will have these symptoms, and even the individuals who have them will discover that they vanish rapidly once the body has completely conformed to their new dieting systems.

Question 10: What sort of liquids would I be able to drink amid low carb Ketogenic diet

Any drink that expands your carb or sugar entrance ought to be maintained a strategic distance from. You can use your espresso with cream, and at times, you can consume red or white wines. However, brew and other unfilled calorie beverages ought to be kept away from. The most vital beverage you ought to consume is water; however you should be careful about natural product smoothies containing some shrouded simple sugars.

Conclusion

Low carb Ketogenic diet has been ended up being practical in offering the body some assistance with maintaining a healthy weight, particularly among the medieval time where antiquated people eat dominatingly meat and fish and they could stay fit, live more, with compelling invulnerability that shields them from a few illnesses and heftiness. In light of this accept and conventions, Ketogenic diet was intended to transform your body into a fat burning mode.

This book has highlighted the advantages of staying with low carb Ketogenic diet, including getting more fit relentlessly and supporting the healthy weight for quite a while. The book has additionally highlighted the straightforward conventionss you ought to take after and, also, a percentage of the best diet formulas and syntheses. You have to remember that the way to an effective weight loss is guaranteeing that you substitute and match whatever number assortments of food parts, as could be expected under the circumstances this will guarantee that you don't get exhausted.

Make sure to check out my other books:

- Beginner's Guide to the Paleo Diet: A Simple Start to Achieving Optimal Health and Weight Loss through the Original Human Diet + 35 FREE RECIPES (FREE)
- Ketogenic Diet: A Beginner's Guide to the Ketogenic Diet (Low Carb, High Fat Diet to Lose Weight and Live a Healthy Lifestyle + 35 Bonus recipes

- <u>Low Carb Diet Recipes: 90 Days of Low Carbohydrate Recipes</u>